The Revolutionary Cannabidiol

By:

Ray Tokes

I0440179

Table of Contents

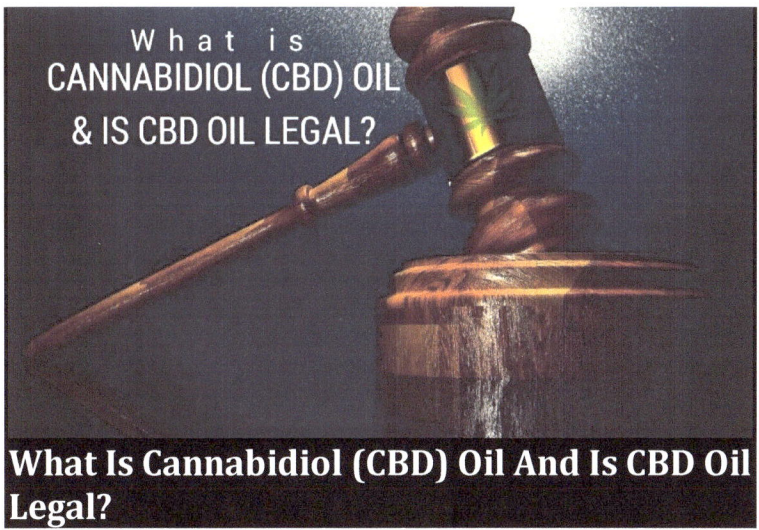

What Is Cannabidiol (CBD) Oil And Is CBD Oil Legal?

Cannabidiol is a compound found in cannabis that is believed to have medical potential without causing the "high" of regular compounds made of marijuana.

Some studies have shown that CBD may counter some of the effects of the psychoactive THC (the chemical that causes a feeling of being high often sought by non-medical users).

Currently around 15 states have legalized marijuana for medical usage.

However more government officials have stated that they were more likely to support a bill legalizing medical use if they could be sure that it wasn't being used to get high.

CBD Oil Legal status depends on who you talk to and where they live as well as where the oil comes from.

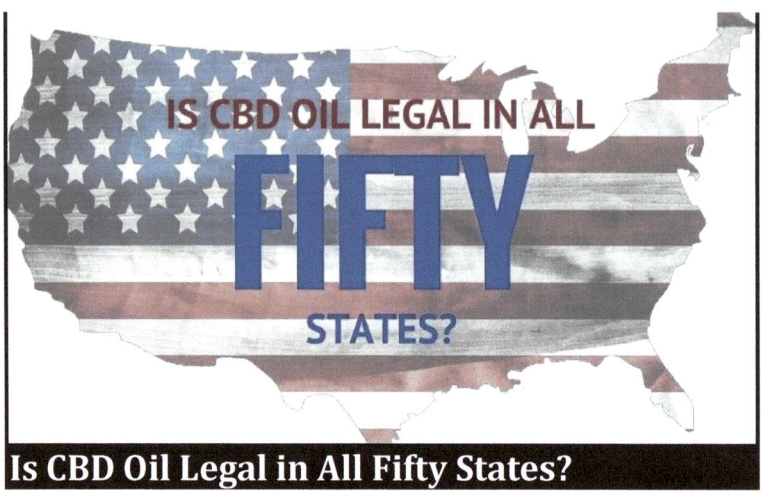

Is CBD Oil Legal in All Fifty States?

Yes, that was read correctly. The source of the CBD Oil is the central question here. CBD made from the marijuana plant is still illegal in most states where marijuana is considered illegal.

However, the Oil when made from hemp is legal in all fifty states according to the DEA.

This is because industrial hemp is legal, and the CBD used for the oil is derived from this plant and not medical marijuana that may continue to have some level of THC in it.

Currently, all legal CBD Oils are produced from hemp in Europe; it's then shipped to Colorado.

From there is sent to all fifty states where consumers can buy it online. This is one of the reasons the cost is so high.

In March 2015, the FDA stated that CBD should be classified as an "unapproved" drug.

Much of the unapproved part is that though some animal studies have found CBD to be useful. Most human studies have been antidotal (subjective evidence made by the consumer).

They insist that more human studies be done to show that the oil does what it's claimed to do.

For this reason, you will want to make sure that your CBD Oil is purchased from a reliable source that measures the amount of both CBD and THC levels.

It's the THC level that could cause it to be considered illegal. It all began in Nov. 2012 when Tikun Olam, an Israeli-based company announced a strain of hemp that contained only CBD as its active ingredient.

One of the more positive aspects of the CBD Oil is that it blocks the receptors needed by THC to work its effects.

Using the oil may reduce the high feeling caused by THC. Of course, this benefit can be seen as a plus or negative.

Most lawmakers consider it a bonus. It allows the oil to be used medically and not recreationally.

Another strong point in favor of the legal version of CBD is that it has no long-term negative side-effects to be considered.

There is also no known level of overdose or death as with most other drugs including alcohol.

This lack of side effects makes it attractive not just to adults but the parents of children with health problems such as epilepsy and ADHD.

All of the drugs used to treat children through medical intervention only have some adverse side effects and could cause death.

There are still some remaining questions about CBD Oils legality.

More human studies are needed to help scientists and doctors understand how and why the oil works as it does. Long-term studies are also necessary to determine if there may not be hidden side-effects.

It's cautioned by many sites that sell the oil that you check the laws of your country and state concerning its use as these rules can be somewhat confusing.

In the US, the FDA has determined the oil to be legal, yet the DEA still treats it as a schedule one drug that must be prescribed and usage monitored.

It's these types of rulings that make it's use so controversial. So be safe and check before buying and buy only from a reputable company to ensure that the product is made from industrial hemp and that no real amount of THC remains in the oil.

Answering Is CBD Oil legal in your state and country can be a little tricky.

The popularity and use of CBD oils and hemp based products is steadily becoming more and more widespread, as people finally begin to understand what these substances actually do to the body and why they can be such a huge benefit to those with debilitating conditions and illnesses.

This is encouraging news, because if CBD oils are ever to be fully utilized alongside treatments for cancer and epilepsy, western societies need to first become comfortable with their public use and the fact that they offer a much healthier alternative to traditional nicotine based products.

With the use, distribution and sale of CBD oils now legal throughout America, it is time for smokers particularly to recognize their many advantages.

Whilst there is still a political and social stigma surrounding the recreational and medical use of marijuana and its derivatives, CBD oils will face an uphill struggle to be accepted.

However, as long as clinical studies continue to produce evidence to support the notion that they can have a significantly positive impact on health, they have a chance to become an effective and successful part of the market.

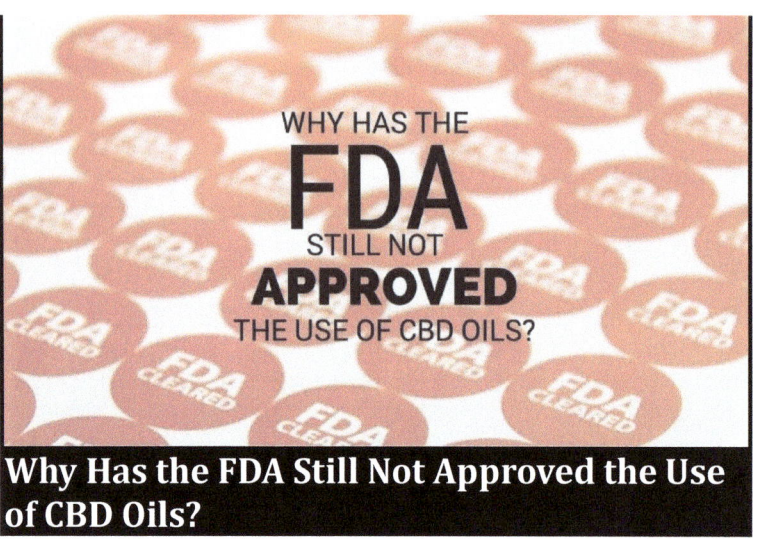

Why Has the FDA Still Not Approved the Use of CBD Oils?

Whilst it is true that the FDA has not yet given its official approval to the use of cannabinoid oils, the truth is that this has less to do with any worries about risk or negative impacts on the mind and body, and more to do with the intricate combination of social, legal, and political factors which push medical industries forward in America, and in other western nations.

There simply has not been enough authorized research into the benefits of CBD at this point, but it does not mean that there will not be more important research conducted in the future.

As long as studies continue to suggest that CBD oil can aid in the fight against ailments like convulsions and inflammation, lessen the suffering related to muscle pain and spasms, and help people suffering from severe illnesses lead a pain free life, there is a good chance that attitudes will continue to change for the better.

At present, CDB oils, vapors, and tinctures cannot be sold to anybody under the age of eighteen years. Once again, this is a decision less related to health factors, and more to do with helping young people resist the temptation to start smoking in the first place.

There is no need to have any kind of special medical permit or license to use CBD oils, vapors or tinctures. However, they are currently only available to customers and vendors resident within the United States.

For those considering an initial foray into 'vaporizing,' the first step is to pick up a high quality vaporizing device (available from all good smoking shops and suppliers) in a flavor which sounds pleasant and appealing.

The typical vaporizer is easy to use, simple to clean and store, and can be carried securely in a pocket, purse, or bag.

It is usually much cheaper to 'smoke' CBD oil vapors than it is to buy and smoke regular cigarettes, so it is also possible to save money by making the switch from nicotine based products to water based hemp oils and cannabis oils.

It is completely legal to smoke CBD oils vapors in public spaces, because they do not produce any harmful emissions or unpleasant odors.

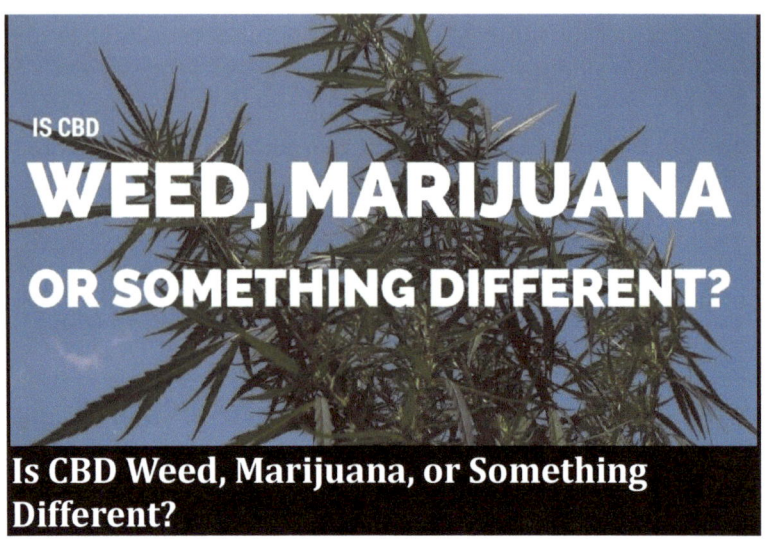

Is CBD Weed, Marijuana, or Something Different?

The confusion surrounding the use of CBD oils seems to stem from the fact that so few people are fully aware of what hemp oil vapors are made from.

This lack of understanding can lead to misplaced fear and anxiety, particularly when it comes to the derivatives of substances which have been partially criminalized, either now or in the past.

As cannabis oil and hemp oil is directly related to the marijuana plant, there are far too many people who wrongly assume that these products are illegal.

The good news is that this is not the case and there is a very good reason why – CBD oil, whilst derived from marijuana, contains none of the psychoactive properties which make the drug illegal.

There is one property in particular (THC) which has a dramatic effect on the brain, and this is why the use of marijuana is criminalized.

However, cannabinoid oils do not contain THC. To be precise, a person cannot get high or significantly alter their mood or mental state by inhaling, smoking, or ingesting cannabis or hemp oils, either as a vapor or a tincture. Yet, CBD oils are believed to have a noticeable effect on the brain, albeit a much milder and safer one than THC.

If a person does swap traditional nicotine cigarettes for CBD oil, they are likely to find that their body feels more relaxed, minor forms of pain are somewhat dulled, and their mood becomes lighter and mellower.

To reiterate, this is not due to the presence of THC, and CBD oils will not get a person high. This should answer issues associated with the question 'Is CBD oil weed, marijuana, or something different?'

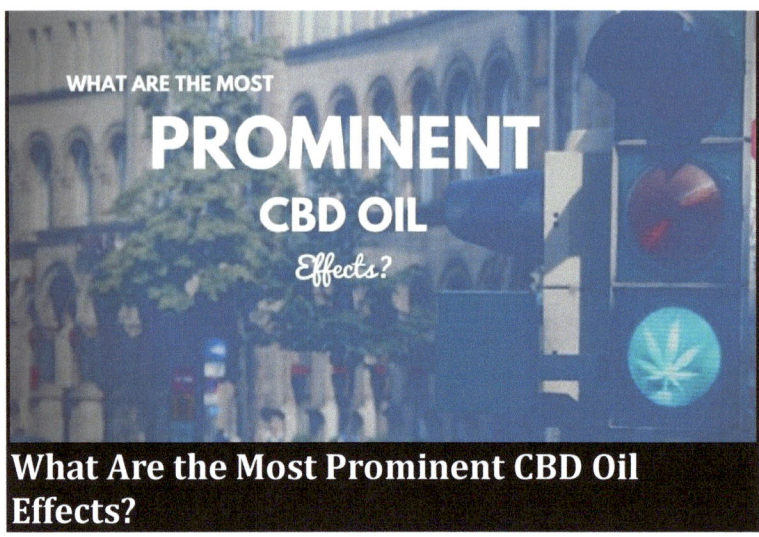

What Are the Most Prominent CBD Oil Effects?

As aforementioned, there are numerous studies which suggest that CBD oil has the power to reduce anxiety levels, help the muscles of the body to relax, and even lessen the sensation of certain kinds of pain and discomfort.

For all of these reasons, hemp oil products and CBD oils are currently in the process of being fully legalized in several countries all around the world.

It is important to point out that the use, sale, and distribution of cannabinoid products (as long as they do not contain THC) is 100% legal in all fifty one US states.

Plus, as far as medical advice goes these days, it is no longer uncommon to hear experts recommend CBD vapors as an effective way to approach kicking a heavy nicotine habit and adapting some of the harmful behaviors associated with smoking.

There is also convincing evidence to suggest that CBD oil (after being extracted from naturally grown hemp) can actively reduce the appearance of aging, make wrinkles less noticeable, and giving sagging skin a significant boost.

For long time nicotine addicts especially, switching to cannabis oils and vapors can be a great way to inject a little extra flexibility and elasticity into the skin.

If years of smoking has wreaked havoc with the complexion, why not think about making a healthy switch to CBD oils and vapors?

It is precisely because CBD oil is most commonly taken into the body using a vaporizer (and that these devices use only water to draw the substances into the lungs), that cannabis oils and vapors are very different to nicotine based cigarettes.

In other words, the lungs are taking in water and not smoke, which is filled with harmful properties when it comes to nicotine and tobacco based products.

This also means that smoking CBD oil with a vaporizer can actually rehydrate the body. If a person needs even more convincing to make the switch from nicotine to CBD oil, they only need to think about the proposed effects on stress and anxiety.

It has been proved, many times, that the behavioral aspects of smoking can be as powerful as the addictive substances themselves.

This means that even puffing on a vaporizer can help calm the nerves and soothe the mind. It is even more advantageous then that hemp oil is believed to have its own relaxing and soothing impact on the mind and body.

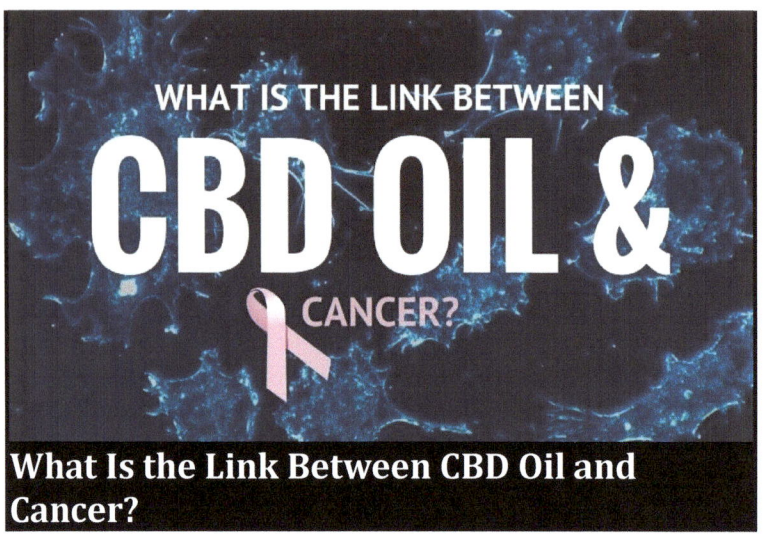

What Is the Link Between CBD Oil and Cancer?

At present, the US Drug Enforcement Administration strictly forbids the possession, prescription, and supply of marijuana based products for recreational use – because they contain THC.

Whilst the distribution, use, and sale of CBD oils (which do not contain THC) are legal across the country, the Food and Drug Administration has not yet given these substances official approval.

It is important to note that this is almost certainly a result of financial and social factors, rather than medical ones.

In fact, there is as yet no evidence to suggest that the medicinal or recreational use of CBD hemp oils has any kind of negative impact on the mind or body.

It is hoped that the FDA will eventually turn their attentions to the official approval of cannabinoid products, perhaps following more extensive scientific research into their benefits.

As for the proposed links between CBD oil and cancer, the evidence is just as murky.

Once again, the problem is not that the evidence for a positive correlation between CBD oil use and the treatment of cancer does not exist, but more that it has not been properly collated or quantified.

It will take a concerted and official (likely state led) investigation into the various benefits of hemp oil products and cannabis derivatives to provide any kind of watertight proof of that it can be used as an effective treatment.

The various different compounds within marijuana are known to provoke different actions from the human body.

For instance, delta-9-tetrahydrocannabinol (or THC) appears to be what causes the well-known 'high' familiar to regular users and believed to have a positive impact on pain relief, nausea, inflammation, and many other conditions and ailments.

According to some experts, it can also be used to treat seizures, lessen anxiety, and regulate mood.

Furthermore, a small number of studies suggest that smoked or vaporized marijuana derivatives may aid with the treatment of neuropathic pain caused by damaged nerves and might even slow down the growth of certain types of cancer cell.

There have been several scientific experiments conducted on animals which have demonstrated a lessened pace of growth (of cancer cells) in a range of small mammals (often mice).

In even more remarkable results, smoking or vaporizing marijuana derivatives is now thought likely to have a positive impact on food intake for HIV sufferers.

Plus, for a long time, medical studies have demonstrated that patients who regularly ingest marijuana extracts actually tend to require significantly less pain medication.

There have been some very important early clinical trials involving cannabinoids when it comes to treating cancer in humans and more studies are planned for the future.

It is important to note that whilst studies have so far suggested that cannabinoids are safe when it comes to treating cancer, they cannot prove that they have the ability to help control or cure the disease.

This means that relying on marijuana or CBD oils, tinctures, or vapors as a primary treatment, whilst avoiding or disregarding conventional medical treatments for cancer, could still have serious health consequences and even result in fatalities.

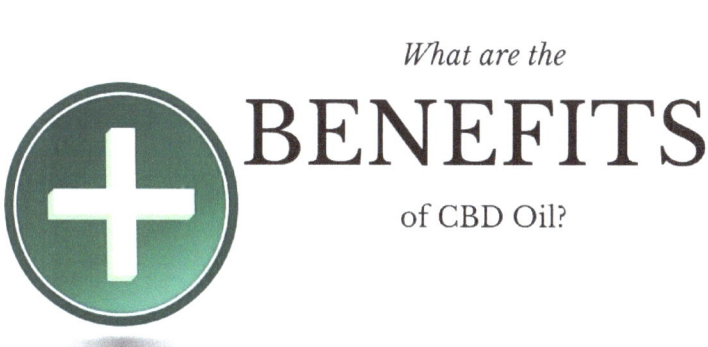

What Are the Benefits of CBD Oil?

CBD Oils Benefits are numerous, for example, it's believed to be useful in Arthritis, anxiety, pain and epilepsy to name just a few of the disorders. Some of the treatment coming from CBD oil is that is an excellent anti-inflammatory.

Today many diseases including heart disease are thought to be triggered by an inflammatory response in the client. It is also possible that the conditions cause the swelling of body tissues affected by the disorder. Regardless of which ends up being found to be true, the fact remains that one of CBD Oil's benefits is that it reduces inflammation in the body.

There is a neat infographic all about CBD.

Another clue can be found in that fact that many of the bodies' organs contain receptors for CBD.

They have been found these receptors in the brain, lungs, liver and immune system just to mention a few.

This information means that the oil may be able to act directly on the organ itself to help correct what's wrong.

Scientists even those who believe that CBD Oil benefits many different illnesses this information is so far just linked to animal studies that may or may not carry over to humans.

They state correctly that most studies must be done on humans. That is the only way to say with certainty that the oil does benefit consumers without long term effects.

Even the most anti-CBD doctors admit that what human studies that have been completed, all show some degree of benefit from the oil. Good news that's accepted at this time is that the lower the dosage, the better the results.

This finding comes from early studies that proved the oil is dose related.

Currently, there is no standard dosing for CBD so if a client is using it without a doctor's advice, they are advised to start low and increase slowly until the disorder is improving.

One of the most studied areas in human usage concerns people; including children do receive some benefit from the drugs ant-convulsion properties.

This statement means that the product significantly reduces seizure activities.

Most of these studies looked at the oils benefits when used with traditional anti-convulsion drugs.

It was found that while both drugs should be taken together to get the greater relief that the conventional drugs may be substantially reduced.

In a few reported cases, the person was able to leave behind the traditional medications.

However, this should not be attempted unless under a medical doctor's care as it could result in death.

One of the types of epilepsy that seems to respond well to CBD Oil's benefits is a type of rare epilepsy called Dravet Syndrome.

This syndrome is a severe and sometimes fatal form of epilepsy that can cause seizures in infants and young children.

Later in life it will make room for other forms of seizure.

This type of epilepsy causes developmental delays as well as other health problems.

It is not easily controlled by traditional medications. It does respond to CBD oil in a big way.

One human study conducted by Stanford University showed that the oil caused a substantial loss of seizures in 84% of the persons in the study.

That is statistically relevant.

It's also though that the oil may lower pain levels. Again most of the studies looked at persons who had chronic pain and took traditional opioids.

The best results were found in people who used both CBD oil and THC. This combination seemed to make opioids work better; meaning fewer were needed to control pain.

This finding could in time reduce the amount of deaths from pain medications. In the US alone that could mean thousands of deaths a year.

Other conditions have seen CDB Oil Benefit such as a reduction in pain from neuron-pathologies such as the type caused by diabetes.

This benefit could help millions of people suffering from this painful disorder. It also seems to help with social anxieties without causing the paranoia seen in THC usage.

CBD oil has been found to be a neuroprotective agent and show promise for use in Alzheimer's and Parkinson's disease.

It also demonstrates that it can reduce the amount of psychosis in patients with Schizophrenia.

To date, the oil does not seem to cure these disorders but rather lessens the symptoms as well if not better than do traditional treatments with medication.

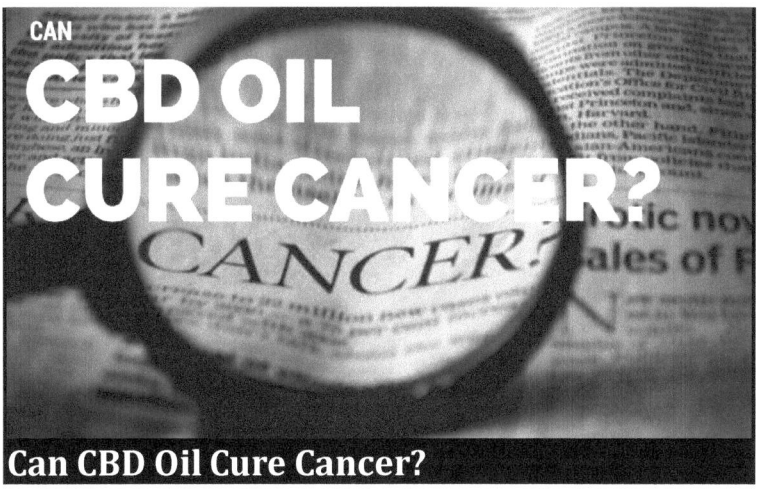

Can CBD Oil Cure Cancer?

Medical Marijuana is thought by some scientists to be a natural form of chemotherapy.

The same seems to hold true for CBD oil.

When used either with or without THC products effects some benefit to most forms of cancer without severe and debilitating side-effects found in most traditional medications used to stop cancer.

It seems to work with many types of cancer though through different mechanisms. Some of the results have been so amazing that doctors in the field have stated that it could cause a major revision in how some cancers are treated.

This change in treatment may be true even of pancreatic cancer, one of the fastest acting malignancies with a very poor cure rate. Many die within months of receiving a diagnosis of pancreatic cancer.

It seems that CBD oil may be proactive against cancer by preventing some forms from ever occurring.

Studies have recently found that persons who used the oil on a regular schedule are 45% less likely to develop bladder cancer than persons not using the oil.

CBD is now thought to be the first non-toxic option for the treatment of invasive forms of cancer such as breast, ovarian and even lung cancer.

How does it do this?

- It triggers cell death in cancerous growths (apoptosis).

- The oil stops cancerous cells from dividing.

- It prevents new blood vessels from forming inside tumors depriving the tumor of needed nutrients.

- It decreases the chance of cancer cells from spreading throughout the body by stopping the cells from entering neighboring cells.

- It can speed up internal waste disposal (known as autophagy), this causes another type of cell death.

Despite claims by the federal government, scientists hired to dispute the claims that CBD oil cures cancer returned a statement saying just that.

Soon, however, they slipped up, and the truth behind the study became common knowledge.

Scientists were working on a different study conducted at the St. George University of London found that CBD weakened the aggression of cancer cells making them much easier to kill with radiation.

Many agree that the compound may become critical in the way we treat glioma (tumors) shortly.

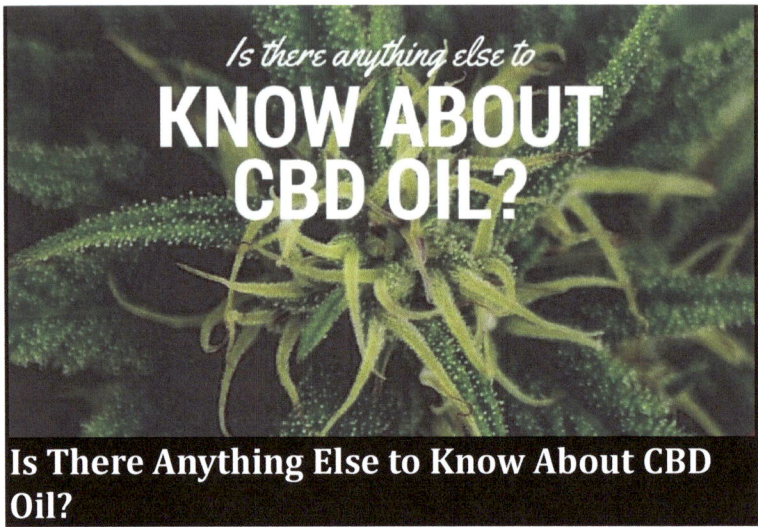

Is There Anything Else to Know About CBD Oil?

While CBD oil is legal in all fifty states of the US, the consumer should still check on laws for their area. There are two types of plants used to make CBD oil.

In the US, the only legal form is produced in Europe and shipped to Colorado and then to all fifty states. Because its widespread acceptance is that the oil contains no THC, so clients don't get high.

It has been found that CBD oil may reduce the likeliness of THC being able to cause a high feeling.

There are many medical studies across the world being conducted on CBD oil.

Most are showing strong promise in the treatment of neuro disorders such as Alzheimer's, Parkinson's and Schizophrenia.

Still its greatest promise comes from it's anti-convulsion properties.

The use of CBD oil in epilepsy is also the most studied field. Other studies have shown that disorders related to inflammation may benefit from the use of CBD oil's anti-inflammatory diseases.

This benefit may include stress and heart disease.

Early studies do seem to support the theory that [CBD oil cures cancer] of all types.

It does so through several different mechanisms. Doctors in the field of oncology (study of cancer) think that it may revolutionize the way all cancers are treated, but more studies are needed.

Currently, the results can only be classified as promising.

As CBD oils do not contain any THC (the property is extracted before sale), there is absolutely no reason why you should not be able to ingest them and still pass a routine drug test.

Whilst there is no nicotine whatsoever in the vast majority of CBD vapors, many do contain nicotine like substances, in order to provide support to individuals who are trying to substitute hemp oils for standard cigarettes.

It is important to understand that this market, whilst a steadily burgeoning one, is also still fairly new.

As it is in its infancy, there are lots of claims about its advantages which are based on a great deal of clinical evidence but have not yet been officially confirmed.

The bottom line is that consumers are really the ones with the power to practically substantiate the benefits of using CBD oils, because they are the ones who are interacting with the products.

For these reasons, it could be argued that the sale of CBD oils and hemp based products is founded on more than just a desire to make profit – the market for nicotine products is one of the most lucrative on the planet, after all.

Rather, the distribution and use of CBD oils is so widely supported, because more and more people are realizing that they can be a viable alternative to harmful and addictive substances like nicotine and tobacco.

Source - http://www.cannabiscbdoil.org

www.ingramcontent.com/pod-product-compliance
Lightning Source LLC
Chambersburg PA
CBHW050928290526
45792CB00002B/936